Ketogenic Diet Book for Beginners

Table of Contents

Additionally, the information in the following pages is intended only for informational purposes and should thus be thought of as universal. As befitting its nature, it is presented without assurance regarding its prolonged validity or interim quality. Trademarks that are mentioned are done without written consent and can in no way be considered an endorsement from the trademark holder.

Introduction

Congratulations on downloading *Ketogenic Diet Book for Beginners* and thank you for doing so. The ketogenic diet is a great way to help jump-start your body's natural fat loss potential and help you to look and feel better than you have in years in the process.

Getting started successfully does require some hard work, however, which is why the following chapters will discuss everything you need to know in order to move forward with this new healthy lifestyle choice successfully. First, you will learn all about what sets the keto diet apart from the pack as well as what you will need in order to follow it yourself. Next, you will learn all about the best ways to get started with keto diet yourself, as well as plenty of tips for dealing with the dreaded keto flu. From there you will find plenty of breakfast, lunch, dinner and snack recipes to help you start off on your new lifestyle choice on the right foot.

There are plenty of books on this subject on the market, thanks again for choosing this one! Every effort was made to ensure it is full of as much useful information as possible, please enjoy!

Chapter 1: Keto Diet Basics

While many different diets are just flash in the pan fads, the ketogenic diet is one that has been around for nearly a century. First developed in the 1920s at the world-famous Mayo Clinic in Minnesota, it was first envisioned as a means to treat patients who were suffering from seizures. Around the same time, the diet was also being explored at the Johns Hopkins medical school in Maryland as a means of dealing with epilepsy in children.

At the time the diet was heralded as an exciting breakthrough when dealing with seizures, though it eventually fell out of fashion when it became possible to deal with seizures with a pill rather than a lifestyle change. The diet ultimately ended up lying fallow for several decades until it was rediscovered by Hollywood film director Jim Abraham who found out about it because his son Charlie was suffering from life-threatening seizures. Thanks to an interview on *Dateline* the world was reminded of the ketogenic diet and it has been gaining popularity ever since.

While there is no doubt that some people still follow a ketogenic lifestyle as a means of dealing with their seizures, a majority of the reason for the continued modern interest in the diet is the science behind how it, and the human body, actually work which wasn't available to the average person in the 1920s. The basics here start with how the average person generates fuel for their body which is by burning glucose that has been stored in the body for energy. Glucose is found in carbohydrates and, much like the food pyramid stated for many decades, a foundational staple of what is known as the Standard American Diet. This diet is high in processed foods as well as carbohydrates, contains a moderate amount of protein and a small number of fats of all types.

Now, when left to its own devices, the human body is perfectly happy burning fat for fuel, this is why excess glucose is converted to fat so it can be used in an emergency. Unfortunately, the high amount of carbs in the Standard American Diet means that it never gets the chance. You see, carbs are far easier to break down for energy than fat is, and the immediate return on the initial invest is higher as well. As such, as long as there are plenty of carbs in the picture the body won't look twice at all of the useful fat that it could be burning instead.

Now, the basis of the ketogenic diet is the state of ketosis which is a natural state the body is capable of dropping into when certain conditions are met. For humanity's ancient ancestors, this meant when they couldn't find enough food to sustain them and their bodies started to starve. Luckily in the 1920s, doctors discovered that this state could also be reached by simply limiting the dieter's intake of carbs to a significant degree. As such, by reducing your net carbohydrate intake to below 15 net grams for anywhere from one to two weeks you can force your body into a ketogenic state.

Once your body reaches ketosis your liver will start to produce ketones which can be broken down for energy.

You can calculate your net carbs by first taking the total number of carbs in a specific product and then subtracting from that its overall fiber content. Once you have started following the keto diet your body will first need to burn through any glucose that is still in its system prior to starting to activate its core ketogenic processes. This will cause the liver to start creating ketones and also breaking down available fat. Breaking down the fat creates two separate molecules, glycerol and fatty acids.

Fatty acid makes the ketogenic process easier to manage for the body by easing the production of ketones and glycerol fills the roll of glucose in scenarios where the body will accept no glucose substitutes. One such instance of this is the brain which use glucose to generate its energy thanks to a process known as gluconeogenesis.

Thus, while you remain in a state of ketosis you can literally expect the fat to melt off your body, albeit fairly slowly if you don't do anything to help it along, starting with the fat found in many traditional problem areas. What's more, the longer your body remains in ketosis the more adept your body will become at burning fat for fuel and the more pronounced the overall effect will become.

Decreases hunger: Beyond simply helping you to burn fat more effectively, following a keto diet is also a great way to lose weight for a number of other reasons, starting with the fact that remaining in ketosis is actually proven to help you to remain feeling full after a meal far longer than would otherwise be the case. This is simply due to the fact that fat is more difficult to process than carbs which means your body won't begin to send out signals saying it is hungry until everything has been completely processed.

Additionally, while you can expect some carb cravings during the early part of ketosis, you will find that after you make it past this hurdle you will be able to remove food from your thoughts more easily than before. This is thanks to a useful hormone known as cholecystokinin which is the natural counter to ghrelin, the hormone responsible for telling you when you are hungry. Cholecystokinin is created by the body when food is moving through the intestines, but if you are in ketosis then it will be created at all times instead. The increased cholecystokinin production will continue for the full time your body remains in a ketogenic state, and even for a few days after you have left it.

Increases natural immunity: Beyond what it can do to your hunger levels, remaining in a ketogenic state is also known to dramatically reduce the likelihood of having to deal with a variety of different health issues, starting with a variety of different types of cancer. While healthy cells can easily burn ketones instead of glucose for fuel, many types of cancer can only feed on glucose which means they would form much more slowly in those who follow the ketogenic diet.

If you are interested in promoting brain health he then keto diet is also right up your alley for a few reasons. The first of these is the fact that it is closer to the way early humans ate, which means it is closer to the type of fuel that the brain has been trained to expect over countless millennia. As such, by following the keto diet you give the brain more of what it wants so that it can do less work for the same amount of benefit.

What's more, while the brain needs glucose to function, too much of a good thing can cause additional issues for those who aren't careful. If the brain receives an extreme amount of glucose for a prolonged period of time it can develop an immunity which will make it have to work harder in order to achieve the same results. Over time, this can lead to issues such as dementia. Ketosis also for the use of glycerol as opposed to glucose which is healthier and will allow it to function properly with less of a chance for degradation to occur at the same time.

Chapter 2: Transitioning to the Keto Diet

While it might seem as though you won't be able to stick with the keto diet at first, the fact of the matter is that the early days of the diet are the most difficult for almost everyone. While the biggest reason for this is the abundance of carbs found in most readily available options, another important reason is that your body has had years and years to get used to breaking down carbs, and very little (if any) experience breaking down fats for energy. As such, it is going to take some time to get these tools up and running.

The period where you won't have enough glucose in your system to power your core bodily systems, while at the same time your body has not yet mange to get ketone production online is known as the keto flu.

Keto flu

During the first seven to 14 days of your new keto lifestyle, you are bound to experience a host of flu-like symptoms. For starters, you are bound to feel tired and sluggish, which is to be expected because your internal batteries will all be hovering around 10 percent. Additionally, you are going to likely feel as though you have a cold, aches, chills, the whole nine yards. What you are actually going to be experiencing is withdrawal, the same as you would when removing any other harmful and addictive substance from your diet. It will all ultimately be worth it, however, as once your body gets with the new program you will be on your way to living the keto lifestyle in perpetuity.

Starting off strong: When you first begin adapting to the ketogenic lifestyle, if you feel as though your body's reaction to the loss of carbs is going to be even more severe than average, or if you have tried once before and found the withdrawal too severe to handle, then you may want to start off by slowly cutting the carbs out of your diet. While this obviously won't provide you with benefits of ketosis, slowly cutting back on your cabs a little bit per week should make the final transition far more manageable.

This doesn't mean it will completely remove all impediments, however, which is why it is important to go in with a proper mindset if you ultimately hope to find success. The keto flu is a necessary part of the process to burn the last of the glucose out of your body, the price of admission if you will. What this means is that if you give into your body's desire for carbs, even for a minute, you will ultimately end up doing yourself more harm than good because a few moments' indiscretion can literally be all it takes to push yourself out of ketosis. A single carb-filled meal can be enough to push you out of ketosis for several days, which will be long enough to force you to have to start the process of surviving the keto flu from scratch.

To make the entire process as manageable as it can be, the first new habit you can start to form is that of drinking more water. Remaining in a ketogenic state is naturally going to leave you more hydrated than would otherwise be the case which means you need to plan on drinking a gallon of water per day. While this might sound like a lot, as long as you keep water by your side throughout the day you will find the goal surprisingly manageable to achieve.

Even better, this will help to fight off the hunger pains you are feeling during the transition period before the body will often mask signals for thirst as signals for hunger if they aren't met quickly enough. If you do still end up feeling hungry it is important to keep in mind that it is really just a carb craving and each hunger pain is really just pushing you closer and closer to ketosis.

Staying the course: While striving to reach ketosis for the first time, it is vital that you stick to no more than 15 net carbs per day. After you have made the transition successfully you can then slowly add back in a net gram of carbs per day, no more than that until you start to see negative results. Everyone's body is different when it comes to the maximum amount of net carbs they can consume per day so once you are well-adapted to the diet you should experiment to find the perfect number for you.

In order to ensure that you are able to successfully stay the course, you are going to want to test your ketone levels every day to ensure they are remaining stable. Luckily, there are numerous different products on the market that can determine such details for you, either by testing your blood or by testing your urine. What these tests check for is a substance known as acetone which is created by the body when a ketone is broken down for energy.

In order to ensure you successfully remain in ketosis indefinitely you are going to want to shoot for a ketone level of 3 which means you are fully in ketosis. If your number rises above 3 then it is a sign that you are not getting enough calories in your diet and you need to make a change ASAP. You can also tell if you are in ketosis if your breath smells like overripe apples and you have a taste a metallic taste on your tongue.

If several days of testing show that you are hanging around the .5 mark then the most likely culprit is the fact that there is too much protein in your diet. Excessive protein ultimately turns to glucose, along with all the problems that come along with it. If you don't feel as though you have much protein to cut out, then you may instead want to add more healthy fats to balance things out in the other direction instead. One great way to get a jump start on extra fat in your diet is by adding a tablespoon of butter and a tablespoon of coconut oil to your morning coffee. This will also help keep you feeling full which can make it easier to get over your lack of early morning carbs.

Avoid grazing: When making the keto diet transition you will likely feel hungrier more regularly as you figure out exactly what works for you when. Regardless, it is important to make a concentrated effort to avoid snacking during this period as it can be an easy way to throw yourself out of ketosis without even realizing what you are doing. When making the keto diet transition you will likely feel hungrier more regularly as you figure out exactly what works for you when. Regardless, it is important to make a concentrated effort to avoid snacking during this period as it can be an easy way to throw yourself out of ketosis without even realizing what you are doing. Likewise, while calories aren't as important to the keto diet as the macros of the foods you are eating, that doesn't mean they can be completely disregarded if you still hope to lose weight. After all, a single serving of any that is 1,000 calories is probably not terribly healthy regardless of how much healthy fat and how few carbs it contains. Overall, it is better to avoid snacking completely while making the transition as your body makes more progress towards ketosis while it's hungry.

Look for healthy, whole foods: When it comes to adapting to the keto lifestyle successfully, it is vital that you take the time to clean out your pantry prior to making the change. It doesn't matter how minor an item, or how much you don't typically care for it if it contains carbs then there will come a point where you will have to force yourself to look the other way. Avoid the battle of wills upfront and remove all temptation early for the best results. In addition to foods that are high in carbs, you are going to want to remove anything processed. Processed foods tend to be much higher in carbs, in addition to a wide variety of artificial additives. This naturally fills most "food" items will lots of filler and leaves little room for healthy lean protein and fats.

While cleaning out your kitchen in preparation for the keto diet is relatively straightforward, finding healthy alternatives can be more difficult to find in certain situations than you might expect. This is due to the unavoidable fact that the marketing trends of the past few decades have made the phrases "low-carb" and "all-natural" practically meaningless. As such, rather than taking a package's word for how healthy it is, you will need to be sure to check out the list of ingredients in order to see for yourself.

If, after taking a closer look, the item in question still seems as though it is something you should put into your system, then odds are you can feel good about eating whatever it is. Likewise, you will want to keep in mind that the types of products that are truly healthy are those that don't need to advertise this fact. The avocado, for example, doesn't need to claim that it is all-natural, you simply know what the average nutritional content is for an avocado, it isn't something that is up for debate. Avoid the hype and stick to natural alternatives for the best results.

Keep it up: Once your body has made it past the keto flu and completely adapted to the keto lifestyle, it is perfectly natural for your weight loss to slow to about one pound per week. It is important to keep in mind that this is not only to be expected, it is the maximum amount of continuous weight loss recommended by healthcare professionals. As such, when your body drops into this cycle, rather than panicking that something is wrong you will want to stay the course to ensure that you stay on the right track. Trying to force your body out of its natural weight loss rhythm is only going to end up causing you more harm than good.

Being aware that the drop off is going to occur will make it easier to avoid the excuse of perceived diminishing returns, thus making it less likely that you will fall back into negative habits as a result and end up negating all of your hard work before you have really had any time to enjoy it. If you feel the temptation to fall back into old habits then you need to keep in mind the amount of time that it took for you to reach your current weight. As this isn't something that happened overnight, it is therefore only reasonable to give yourself the same amount of time to make a meaningful change.

Likewise, you will need to keep in mind that as you get closer to your ideal weight your weight loss will continue to slow as your body is closer to its equilibrium as your body will have to do more work to see the same results. Likewise, it is perfectly natural to hit weight loss plateaus from time to time when you won't lose any weight for a week or more. This too is just part of the process and using it as an excuse to slip out of ketosis, even for a few days, will do nothing to improve the issue and only leave you worse off than when you started.

Instead, it is important to take these potential setbacks in stride so that you aren't tempted to use them as an excuse to fall back into bad habits. Never forget, the keto diet will give you the results you need in time, all you need to do is stick with it.

Exercise more

While dealing with the keto flu can make it difficult to do much of anything, studies show that high intensity cardio and body weight exercises during this time can help you to reach ketosis as quickly as possible. This is because these types of exercises are the ones that haven been proven to help your body fly through its stockpile of carbs as quickly as can be. This will ensure that it has no choice but to start burning fat in as little time as possible.

What follows are a number of carb-burning exercise routines that have been specifically designed for various levels of fitness. When you are getting started it is also important to keep in mind that your body is currently operating on far less fuel than it is used to which means you need to be on the lookout for signs of fatigue and don't push yourself past a safe point.

10-minute workout

You will want to repeat the following exercises three times, with a 10 second breather in between. Try and ensure each set of exercises doesn't take more than 3 minutes total.

Jab, cross, front kick (left): Start with your left foot in front of your right foot and your hips facing right. Raise your arms so that you are in somewhat of a boxer stance. Start with a jab by punching forward with your left arm straight out. Move directly into throwing a cross by punching with your left arm and rotating your body to the right. This should leave the full weight of your body on your right foot and your right heel should raise slightly off of the floor. End the sequence by kicking forward with your back foot.

Jab, cross front kick (right): The same as above but in reverse.

Jumping jacks: This exercise is great for improving coordination as well as increasing blood flow. Start with your feet together and arms at your sides before jumping and spreading your arms and your feet before returning to the starting position. To enhance the difficulty, add in a torso twist when you jump.

Sumo squats: Start with your feet at slightly more than hip-width apart and keep your toes pointed facing outward at a 45-degree angle. Place all of your weight on the heels of your feet, your chest upright and your back straight, lower yourself down towards the ground until your thighs are essentially parallel to the ground. Using your quads and your glutes, push yourself back into the starting position. To end each set, move into a reverse lung and fold your body forward while keeping your arms stretched overhead.

20-minute workout

Move through the following exercises three times, allow yourself 15 minutes between sets.

Coffee grinder kick-ups: To begin this exercise start in a squatting position before lifting one leg into the air while resting the entirety of your weight on the other leg. Next, move the leg in the air towards the front of the body in a circular motion. When your two legs get close to one another place your hands in front of you on the floor and force yourself off the ground for a moment so the rotating leg can move past. Shift your weight back to your other leg and repeat the process. Consider each full rotation to be a single repetition. This exercise benefits the legs and the core.

Butt kickers: Jog in place, extending your leg at the back of your stride so that your heel strikes your butt.

Squats: Start in a relaxed position with your feet directly beneath your hips. Raise your hands so they are parallel to the floor and slowly lower yourself towards the floor as far as possible before returning to the starting position. Repeat as many times as possible.

Double toe tap: To begin this exercise you will want to get into a plank position, ensuring your weight is on your forearms and your feet are touching. From there you will want to tense your core and, while keeping your back straight, spread your legs and tap each foot on the group before returning it to the original position. Keep in mind that this exercise requires a fair degree of balance so you may want to take things slow at first. This exercise is useful in strengthening the legs along with the core.

Triceps back dips: To begin this exercise you will want to find a low bench to support yourself against. You will then want to face away from the bench and place your hands directly behind you so they are resting on the bench. Stretch your legs out in front of you with your feet touching one another and then, using your arms, lower yourself towards the ground as far as you can without losing your balance. Keep your elbows tight at your sides as you do each repetition and focus more on form than on hitting a predetermined target. This exercise is useful in strengthening the back as well as the shoulders.

30-minute workout

Mix and match seven of the exercises outlined above and repeat the process three times, allowing yourself 15 seconds to rest in between.

Chapter 3: Breakfast Recipes

Keto breakfast sandwich

Total Prep & Cooking Time: 10 minutes

Yields: 2 Servings

Nutrition Facts (per serving)

- Protein: 16 grams

- Net Carbs: 2 grams

- Fats: 25.3 grams

- Calories: 301

What to Use

- Pepper (as desired)

- Salt (as desired)

- Tabasco (as desired)

- Eggs (4 large)

- Deli ham (.25 oz.)

- Provolone cheese (2 oz. thick slices)

- Coconut oil (2 T)

What to Do

- Add the oil to the pan before placing it on the stove over a burner turned to a medium heat. Add in the eggs and allow them to reach your desired level of doneness.

- Using the eggs as the base of your sandwich, add in the rest of your ingredients as desired.

- Season as desired prior to serving.

Bacon, eggs and avocado

Total Prep & Cooking Time: 12 minutes

Yields: 4 Servings

Nutrition Facts (per serving)

- Protein: 8 grams

- Net Carbs: 1 grams

- Fats: 14 grams

- Calories: 208

What to Use

- Pepper (as desired)

- Salt (as desired)

- Bacon strips (4)

- Eggs (2 large)

- Avocado (.5 sliced)

- Coconut oil (2 T)

What to Do

- In a large saucepan, add in the eggs before filling the pan with enough water that the eggs are submerged under 1 inch of water.

- Add the pan to the stove over a saucepan turned to a high heat. After the water boils, remove the pan from the stove and let the contents cool for 12 minutes.

- Ensure your oven is heated to 350F

- Peel the eggs and cut them in half vertically.

- Add the yolks to a mixing bowl and mash well.

- Add the bacon to a baking sheet before placing the sheet in the oven for about 5 minutes. Remove the bacon from the oven and crumble.

- Add the avocado the bowl with the egg yolk and mass the two together until they are blended well. Season as desired before adding in the crushed bacon and mixing well.

- Scoop the results in to the eggs and serve.

Omelet with mushrooms

Total Prep & Cooking Time: 15 minutes

Yields: 1 Serving

Nutrition Facts (per serving)

- Protein: 21 grams

- Net Carbs: 4 grams

- Fats: 34.6 grams

- Calories: 401

What to Use

- Pepper (as desired)

- Salt (as desired)

- Coconut oil (2 T)

- Eggs (3 large)

- Cheddar cheese (1 oz. shredded)

- Yellow onion (.25)

- Mushrooms (3)

-

What to Do

- Add the oil to the pan before placing it on the stove over a burner turned to a medium heat.

- Place the eggs in a mixing bowl before whisking well and seasoning as needed.

- Add the eggs to the skillet before allowing them to cook a few minutes until the bottom is firm and the top is raw.

- Mix in the remaining ingredients before folding the omelet in half with the help of a spatula. You will know it has finished cooking when the bottom of the omelet is golden brown.

Breakfast sandwich with avocado

Total Prep & Cooking Time: 15 minutes

Yields: 1 Serving

Nutrition Facts (per serving)

- Protein: 15 grams

- Net Carbs: 1.3 grams

- Fats: 26.4 grams

- Calories: 333

What to Use

- Pepper (as desired)

- Salt (as desired)

- Coconut oil (2 T)

- Sausage patties (2)

- Egg (1 medium)

- Cream cheese (1 T)

- Cheddar cheese (2 T)

- Avocado (.25 sliced)

What to Do

- Add the oil to the pan before placing it on the stove over a burner turned to a medium/high heat. Place the sausage in the pan and allow it to cook for 60 seconds per side. Remove the sausage from the pan while retaining the grease.

- Place all of the cheese into a bowl that is microwave safe and then microwave it on full power for 30 seconds. Mix well.

- Place the eggs in the greasy pan and allow them to cook until the bottom is firm but the top is relatively raw.

- Add in the remaining omelet ingredients before then using the spatula to fold the omelet in half. You will be able to tell the omelet is finished cooking when the bottom is a golden brown.

- Remove the omelet from the pan and place it between the two sausage patties.

- Serve and enjoy!

Pancakes

Total Prep & Cooking Time: 11 minutes

Yields: 4 Servings

Nutrition Facts (per serving)

- Protein: 11.2 grams

- Net Carbs: 2.4 grams

- Fats: 20 grams

- Calories: 234

What to Use

- Coconut oil (2 T)

- Almond flour (.5 c + 1 T)

- Cream cheese (.5 c)

- Eggs (4 large)

- Cinnamon (.5 tsp.)

- Erythritol (1 tsp. optional)

What to Do

- Add the oil to the pan before placing it on the stove over a burner turned to a medium/high heat.

- Mix all of the ingredients together in a blender and blend until smooth.

- Place 25 percent of the batter into the pan so that it forms a pancake shape. Cook each pancake about 1 minute per side.

Eggs, avocado and bacon

Total Prep & Cooking Time: 25 minutes

Yields: 2 Servings

Nutrition Facts (per serving)

- Protein: 12 grams

- Net Carbs: 5.2 grams

- Fats: 26.2 grams

- Calories: 321

What to Use

- Pepper (as desired)

- Salt (as desired)

- Avocado (1)

- Eggs (2 large)

- Bacon (1 slice)

- Sharp cheddar cheese (1 T shredded)

What to Do

- Add the oil to the pan before placing it on the stove over a burner turned to a medium/high heat.

- Ensure your over is set to 425F.

- Add the bacon to the pan and fry well before adding in the spinach.

- While the spinach cooks slice the avocado before removing the skin and the pit. Place the halves of the avocado into a muffin tin to cook.

- Add the remaining ingredients to the avocado halves, taking care to use the egg as a base.

- After placing the muffin tin in the oven allow the avocado to cook about 15 minutes.

Chia seed pudding

Total Prep & Cooking Time: 10 minutes

Yields: 2 Servings

Nutrition Facts (per serving)

- Protein: 10 grams

- Net Carbs: 1 grams

- Fats: 23 grams

- Calories: 223

What to Use

- Blueberries (1.4 o.)

- Chia seeds (6 T)

- Coconut milk (2 c)

- Vanilla extract (.5 tsp.)

- Maple syrup (1 T)

What to Do

- Add everything but the blueberries to a jar before placing a lid on it and shaking everything well for about 30 seconds.

- Allow the pudding to stand for about 5 minutes before shaking another 30 seconds. Wait another 5 minutes and repeat.

- Retire the jar to the refrigerator to allow it to set for about 2 hours.

- Add in the blueberries and mix well prior to serving.

Keto hash browns

Total Prep & Cooking Time: 45 minutes

Yields: 3 Servings

Nutrition Facts (per serving)

- Protein: 18 grams

- Net Carbs: 3.8 grams

- Fats: 31 grams

- Calories: 361

What to Use

- Pepper (as desired)

- Coconut oil (2 T)

- Salt (as desired)

- Cauliflower (1 head)

- Eggs (2 large)

- Scallions (1 bunch, diced)

- Ham (8 oz. chopped)

- Sharp cheddar (3 T shredded)

What to Do

- Take a cheese grater to the cauliflower florets and add the results to a mixing bowl before adding in the eggs, scallions, ham, coconut oil, cheese and any desired seasonings before mixing well.

- Take .5 c of the mixture and add it to a warm waffle iron and allow the hash brown to cook until it is golden brown.

- You will need to remove it from the waffle iron gently lest it break.

Keto Bagel

Total Prep & Cooking Time: 29 minutes

Yields: 6 Servings

Nutrition Facts (per serving)

- Protein: 27.8 grams
- Net Carbs: 6 grams
- Fats: 35 grams
- Calories: 449

What to Use

- Pepper (as desired)
- Coconut oil (2 T)
- Salt (as desired)
- Everything bagel seasoning (3 T)
- Cream cheese (5 To
- Mozzarella cheese (3 c shredded)
- Eggs (3 large, divided)
- Italian seasoning (1 tsp.)
- Onion powder (1 tsp.)
- Garlic powder (1 tsp.)

- Baking powder 91 T)

- Almond flour (2 c)

What to Do

- Ensure your over is set to 425F.

- In a mixing bowl, Italian seasoning, almond flour, baking powder, garlic powder and onion powder and mix well.

- Separately, whisk one of the eggs.

- In a third, microwave safe bowl combine the mozzarella cheese and cream cheese. Microwave the bowl for 90 seconds and mix again. Microwave an additional 60 seconds and mix again.

- Add in the other two eggs to the bowl of flour and combine everything until it is well incorporated. If the dough becomes unmanageable you can microwave it for 30 seconds to get it under control.

- Split the dough into six sections and roll each into a ball before poking your finger through each to form a hole.

- Place each finished bagel onto a prepared baking sheet before using some egg to brush the top of each bagel. Top with everything bagel seasoning and then place the baking sheet in the oven for about 12 minutes.

- Top each bagel with approximately 4 oz. of the mixed cream cheese prior to serving.

Denver Omelet

Total Prep & Cooking Time: 45 minutes

Yields: 6 Servings

Nutrition Facts (per serving)

- Protein: 12 grams
- Net Carbs: 6 grams
- Fats: 28.5 grams
- Calories: 398

What to Use

- Pepper (as desired)
- Coconut oil (2 T)
- Salt (as desired)
- Cheddar cheese (.5 c shredded)
- Milk (.3 c)
- Eggs (8 large)
- Ham (1 c cooked)
- Yellow onion (.3 c)
- Red bell pepper (1 c)

What to Do

- Ensure your over is set to 400F.

- Add the oil to the pan before placing it on the stove over a burner turned to a medium/high heat. Add in the peppers and onions and allow them to cook about 4 minutes until everything has softened.

- Add everything to the baking dish and use it to form a layer above the ham.

- In a mixing bowl, combine the eggs and the milk and mix well. Season as needed before adding to the baking dish.

- Place the baking dish in the oven for about 23 minutes or until it is puffy and risen.

- Allow the omelet to cool 5 minutes prior to serving.

Egg muffins

Total Prep & Cooking Time: 25 minutes

Yields: 4 Servings

Nutrition Facts (per serving)

- Protein: 18 grams

- Net Carbs: 2 grams

- Fats: 38 grams

- Calories: 356

What to Use

- Pepper (as desired)

- Salt (as desired)

- Eggs (6 large)

- Scallion (1 chopped)

- Bacon (5 oz.)

- Cheese (3 oz. shredded)

- Green pesto (1 T)

What to Do

- Ensure your over is set to350F.

- Add the oil to the pan before placing it on the stove over a burner turned to a medium/high heat. Once the pan has warmed, add in the bacon and let it cook until it is crispy.

- Place the eggs into a mixing bowl and whisk them along with the pesto and the seasonings.

- Crumble the bacon and it to the mixing bowl along with the cheese and combine thoroughly.

- Add the mixture evenly to 4 of the 6 cups of a muffin tin and then place them in the oven for about 15 minutes. You will know they are ready when you can stick a toothpick through the center one and pull it out cleanly.

Egg scramble

Total Prep & Cooking Time: 15 minutes

Yields: 4 Servings

Nutrition Facts (per serving)

- Protein: 8 grams

- Net Carbs: 2 grams

- Fats: 22.1 grams

- Calories: 287

What to Use

- Pepper (as desired)

- Coconut oil (2 T)

- Salt (as desired)

- Eggs (6 large)

- Scallion (1 chopped)

- Jalapenos (2 finely chopped)

- Tomato (1 finely chopped)

- Sharp cheddar (3 oz.)

What to Do

- Add the oil to the pan before placing it on the stove over a burner turned to a medium/high heat. Once the oil has melted, add in the tomato, jalapenos, and scallions and allow them to cook about 3 minutes.

- While the vegetables are frying, add the eggs to a small bowl and beat them well prior to adding them to the pan.

- Scramble the eggs about 2 minutes until they reach your desired consistency and top with cheese prior to serving.

Eggs, tomatoes and bacon

Total Prep & Cooking Time: 45 minutes

Yields: 6 Servings

Nutrition Facts (per serving)

- Protein: 9 grams

- Net Carbs: 1 grams

- Fats: 22 grams

- Calories: 302

What to Use

- Pepper (as desired)

- Coconut oil (2 T)

- Salt (as desired)

- Eggs (8 medium)

- Bacon (5.3 oz.)

- Cherry tomatoes (2 sliced)

- Parsley (2 T)

What to Do

- Ensure your over is set to 400F.

- Add the oil to the pan before placing it on the stove over a burner turned to a medium/high heat. Once the oil has melted, add in the bacon and fry it as desired.

- Once you have finished cooking the bacon you will want to remove it from the pan while retaining the grease. Add the eggs to the pan, along with the tomatoes, and cook until the eggs reach your desired level of doneness.

- Season as desired and plate with parsley.

Keto porridge

Total Prep & Cooking Time: 15 minutes

Yields: 1 Serving

Nutrition Facts (per serving)

- Protein: 1.8 grams

- Net Carbs: 4 grams

- Fats: 20 grams

- Calories: 240

What to Use

- Coconut cream (4 T)

- Salt (1 pinch)

- Psyllium husk (1 pinch powdered)

- Coconut milk (as desired)

- Butter (1 oz.)

- Egg (1 large)

- Coconut flour (1 T)

What to Do

- With the exception of the coconut milk, add all of the ingredients to a saucepan and combine thoroughly. Place the saucepan on top of a burner that has been turned to a low heat. Stir as desired to achieve preferred consistency.

- Add the coconut milk as desired.

Frittata with Spinach

Total Prep & Cooking Time: 40 minutes

Yields: 4 Servings

Nutrition Facts (per serving)

- Protein: 17 grams

- Net Carbs: 4 grams

- Fats: 24.4 grams

- Calories: 375

What to Use

- Pepper (as desired)

- Coconut oil (2 T)

- Salt (as desired)

- Eggs (8 large)

- Heavy whipping cream (1 c)

- Spinach (8 oz.)

- Bacon (5.3 oz.)

- Sharp cheddar (5.3 oz.)

What to Do

- Ensure your over is set to 350F.

- Add the oil to the pan before placing it on the stove over a burner turned to a medium/high heat. Allow the oil to melt before adding in the bacon and letting it fry until crispy before adding in the spinach.

- In a small mixing bowl, combine the heavy whipping cream and eggs and whisk well.

- Add the results to a prepared baking dish before crumbling the bacon and adding it, the cheese and the egg to the mixture and combining thoroughly.

- Place the dish in the oven and let it bake for approximately 25 minutes.

- Let cool 5 minutes prior to serving.

Avocado Smoothie

Total Prep & Cooking Time: 5 minutes

Yields: 1 Serving

Nutrition Facts (per serving)

- Net Carbs: 6 grams

- Protein: 26 grams

- Fats: 38 grams

- Calories: 587

What to Use

- Unsweetened coconut milk (1 c)

- Avocado (.5)

- Chia seeds (1 T)

- Whey protein powder (1 scoop)

- Gelatin (.5 T)

- Stevia (as desired)

- Coconut oil (2 T)

- Ice cubes (5)

- Cacao nibs (1.5 T)

What to Do

- To create a thicker smoothie you are going to want to start the preparations the night before by combining the chia seeds and the coconut milk and mix well. Stir multiple times over a three hour window and then all the mixture to sit overnight.

- When you are prepared to make your smoothie you will want to slice your avocado prior to removing the seeds and skin. Add all of the ingredients, save the ice and coconut oil, to a blender and blend well.

- Add in the coconut oil and ensure it is incorporated well.

- Finally, add in the ice and blend until it reaches your desired level of thickness. Take care to add the ice last for a smoother, creamier smoothie.

Chapter 4: Lunch Recipes

Pizza Chicken

Total Prep & Cooking Time: 45 minutes

Yields: 6 Servings

Nutrition Facts (per serving)

- Protein: 25 grams
- Net Carbs: 6 grams
- Fats: 38 grams
- Calories: 492

What to Use

- Chicken breast (1 lb.)
- Pizza sauce (.5 c)
- Pizza seasoning (1.5 T)
- Mozzarella cheese (4 oz.)
- Pepperoni (2 oz.)
- Broccoli (2 c steamed)

What to Do

- Ensure your over is set to 375F.

- Place the chicken on a baking sheet before rubbing it down thoroughly with the pizza seasoning. Cover the chicken in pizza sauce before placing it in the oven for about 8 minutes.

- Remove the chicken from the oven before topping with pepperoni and cheese.

- Return the chicken to the oven for another 6 minutes or until its internal temperature reaches 165F.

- Plate with steamed broccoli prior to serving.

Zoodle Lasagna

Total Prep & Cooking Time: 45 minutes

Yields: 4 Servings

Nutrition Facts (per serving)

- Protein: 34 grams

- Net Carbs: 4 grams

- Fats: 41 grams

- Calories: 544

What to Use

- Ground beef (16 oz.)

- Low-carb marinara sauce (1 c)

- Zucchini (1 large)

- Ricotta cheese (10 oz.)

- Mozzarella cheese (4 oz.)

What to Do

- Ensure your over is set to 350F.

- Peel the zucchini and then continue to use the peeler so that you form long strips of zucchini while watching out for the seeds near the core. Salt the zoodles and let them sit for 15 minutes before using a paper towel to remove any left over moisture.

- Place the ground beef in a skillet before placing the skillet on the stove over a burner turned to a medium/high heat. Season the meat as desired prior to adding in the low-carb marinara sauce.

- Once the meat has browned, place half of it in a small casserole dish, followed by half of the zoodles and then half of the meat. Repeat this process once more so the cheese ends up on top.

- Using tinfoil, cover the casserole dish and place the lasagna in the oven for about 30 minutes.

- Remove the lasagna from the oven and prepare your broiler. Broil the lasagna for about 3 minutes to give the cheese time to brown.

- Let the lasagna sit 5 minutes before serving.

Lemon chicken with asparagus

Total Prep & Cooking Time: 30 minutes

Yields: 4 Servings

Nutrition Facts (per serving)

- Protein: 12 grams
- Net Carbs: 5 grams
- Fats: 18.7 grams
- Calories: 183

What to Use

- Pepper (as desired)
- Coconut oil (2 T)
- Salt (as desired)
- Chicken breast (4 skinless, boneless)
- Tapioca flour (.25 c)
- Asparagus stalks (1 lb.)
- Garlic (2 cloves crushed)
- Lemon juice (3 T)
- Lemon zest (1 tsp.)
- Dijon mustard (1 T)
- Chicken stock (1 c)

What to Do

- Place each of the chicken breasts between two pieces of plastic wrap and pound them until they are proximately .25 inches thick.

- Mix together salt, flour and pepper in a mixing bowl before placing the chicken in the bowl and mixing well.

- Add 1 T oil to the pan before placing it on the stove over a burner turned to a medium/high heat. After the oil has warmed up, add in the chicken and cook it for about 5 minutes per side or until its internal temperature reaches 165F. Remove the chicken from the pan prior to cooking the asparagus.

- Add the remaining oil to the pan before adding in the stalks of asparagus and letting them cook for about a minute before adding in the garlic and cooking an additional 60 seconds.

- While the asparagus is cooking, add the lemon juice and Dijon mustard to a small cup and mix well.

- Add the mixture to the pan before turning the heat to high and allowing everything to boil. After it boils, reduce the heat and allow it the pan to simmer about 3 minutes or until the asparagus becomes tender.

- Plate the asparagus and top with the chicken before drizzling with excess liquid.

Brussels sprouts and chicken

Total Prep & Cooking Time: 35 minutes

Yields: 2 Servings

Nutrition Facts (per serving)

- Protein: 16 grams
- Net Carbs: 4 grams
- Fats: 28.6 grams
- Calories: 564

What to Use

- Pepper (as desired)
- Coconut oil (2 T)
- Salt (as desired)
- Brussels sprouts (.5 lbs. sliced)
- Chicken breasts (2)
- Spicy mustard (.25 c)
- Lemon juice (1 T)
- Thyme (1 tsp.)

What to Do

- In a small ramekin, add the seasonings, spicy mustard, lemon juice and thyme and whisk well to combine thoroughly.

- Place the chicken into a large Ziploc bag before adding in the mustard mixture and shaking well to ensure the chicken is well-coated. Allow the chicken to marinate for at least 1 hour.

- Ensure your over is set to 350F.

- Prepare a baking sheet by covering it with parchment paper.

- Add the sliced brussels sprouts into a bowl before coating with coconut oil and then topping with a salt and pepper mixture as desired.

- Place the coated brussels sprouts on the baking sheet to form a single layer.

- Place the chicken in a glass baking pan and then place it in the oven for about 10 minutes. At this point place the baking sheet in the oven as well and cook everything for an additional 15 minutes or until the chicken reaches an internal temperature of 165F.

Avocado and tuna salad

Total Prep & Cooking Time: 20 minutes

Yields: 4 Servings

Nutrition Facts (per serving)

- Protein: 15.6 grams

- Net Carbs: 4.2 grams

- Fats: 21.5 grams

- Calories: 266

What to Use

- Pepper (as desired)

- Coconut oil (2 T)

- Salt (as desired)

- Tuna (15 oz., drained, flaked)

- Cucumber (1 sliced)

- Avocados (2 large, peeled, sliced, pitted)

- Red onion (1 small, thinly sliced)

- Cilantro (.25 c chopped)

- Lemon juice (2 T)

What to Do

- In a salad bowl, combine all of the ingredients, save the lemon juice and oil and toss to combine thoroughly.

- Separately, mix together 2 T lemon juice, 2 T coconut oil, 1 tsp. salt and .25 tsp. pepper and whisk well.

- Add the dressing to the salad and toss to coat prior to serving.

Enchilada bowl

Total Prep & Cooking Time: 20 minutes

Yields: 4 Servings

Nutrition Facts (per serving)

- Protein: 18 grams

- Net Carbs: 5.1 grams

- Fats: 22 grams

- Calories: 240

What to Use

- Pepper (as desired)

- Coconut oil (2 T)

- Salt (as desired)

- Chicken breasts (2, portioned into 4 pieces)

- Enchilada sauce (.75 c red sauce)

- Water (.25 c)

- Onion (.25 c)

- Green chilies (4 oz.)

- Cauliflower rice (12 oz.)

- Avocado (1 chopped)

What to Do

- Add the oil to the pan before placing it on the stove over a burner turned to a medium heat. Add in the enchilada sauce, chilies, onion and water and then reduce the heat to allow everything to simmer, covered, until the chicken is fully cooked and has an internal temperature of 165F.

- After the chicken has cooked, remove it from the pan and shred it before adding it back into the sauce. Allow everything to simmer another 10 minutes, uncovered.

- Plate the cauliflower rice and the chicken and serve with avocado.

Stuffed avocado

Total Prep & Cooking Time: 30 minutes

Yields: 3 Servings

Nutrition Facts (per serving)

- Protein: 22 grams

- Net Carbs: 2.2 grams

- Fats: 31 grams

- Calories: 326

What to Use

- Pepper (as desired)

- Keto mayo (.3)

- Salt (as desired)

- Chicken breasts (2)

- Bacon (3 strips)

- Avocado (2)

- Grape tomatoes (.3 c chopped)

What to Do

- Season the chicken as desired before placing it on a warm grill and cooking until it reaches an internal temperature of 165 degrees.

- Crumble the bacon and cube the chicken before adding them both to a bowl along with the grape tomatoes and keto mayo and combining thoroughly.

- Slice the avocados in halve and remove the pit before filling each half with the chicken mixture.

- Serve and enjoy!

Bok choy, mushrooms and salmon

Total Prep & Cooking Time: 30 minutes

Yields: 4 Servings

Nutrition Facts (per serving)

- Protein: 20.6 grams

- Net Carbs: 4.1 grams

- Fats: 35 grams

- Calories: 527

What to Use

- Pepper (as desired)

- Coconut oil (2 T)

- Salt (as desired)

- Salmon fillet (4)

- Portobello mushrooms (2 caps)

- Bok choy (4)

- Sesame seeds (1 T toasted)

- Green onion (.5)

- Sesame oil (1 tsp.)

- Coconut aminos (1 T)

- Ginger (.5 in. grated)

- Lemon juice (.5 lemon)

What to Do

- In a small mixing bowl, combine the coconut oil, coconut aminos, sesame oil, lemon juice, ginger, .5 tsp. salt and .5 tsp. pepper and whisk well.

- Add half of the marinade to the salmon and ensure it is well-coated. Cover the fish and then allow it to sit in the refrigerator for a minimum of 1 hour.

- Ensure your over is set to 400F.

- Trim the bok choy before cutting it in half and then slicing the mushrooms into half-inch pieces. Top with the rest of the marinade and toss well before adding the results to a prepared baking sheet. Don't forget to leave room for the salmon.

- Place the salmon on the baking sheet with the skin facing down. Place the fish in the oven for about 20 minutes or until the fish starts to flake easily if you touch it with a fork.

Thai chicken with a kick

Total Prep & Cooking Time: 15 minutes

Yields: 4 Servings

Nutrition Facts (per serving)

- Protein: 25 grams

- Net Carbs: 5.1 grams

- Fats: 31.6 grams

- Calories: 298

What to Use

- Pepper (as desired)

- Coconut oil (2 T)

- Salt (as desired)

- Chicken (1 lb. ground)

- Red curry paste (2 T)

- Ginger (1 T minced)

- Garlic (4 cloves minced)

- Red bell pepper (.25 sliced thin)

- Green onions (.5 chopped)

- Coleslaw mix (.25 c)

- Hoisin sauce (.25 c)

- Basil (3 T chopped)

What to Do

- Add the oil to the pan before placing it on the stove over a burner turned to a medium/high heat. Place the chicken in the pan and allow it to brown prior to breaking it up using a wooden spoon.

- Add in the red curry paste, garlic, coleslaw and peppers and allow everything to cook about 3 minutes before adding in the hoisin sauce and green onions and tossing to combine.

- Remove the skillet from the burner, add the basil and toss.

Bacon bratwurst

Total Prep & Cooking Time: 25 minutes

Yields: 4 Servings

Nutrition Facts (per serving)

- Protein:28 grams
- Net Carbs: 2.6 grams
- Fats: 34 grams
- Calories: 507

What to Use

- Beer (24 oz.)
- Bacon (4 slices)
- Romaine lettuce (4 leaves)
- Cheese (4 slices)
- Salt (as desired)
- Pepper (as desired)
- Bratwurst (4)

What to Do

- Pour the beer into a pan prior to adding in the bratwurst and setting it on top of a burner turned to a high heat. Allow them to cook, covered for about 10 minutes.

- After removing each bratwurst from the pan, wrap each in bacon.

- Place the bratwurst on a grill that has been preheated and grill each until the bacon is crisp.

- Wrap each bacon bratwurst in lettuce prior to serving.

Pinwheels

Total Prep & Cooking Time: 30 minutes

Yields: 5 Servings

Nutrition Facts (per serving)

- Protein: 16.7 grams

- Net Carbs: 1.2 grams

- Fats: 16.8 grams

- Calories: 620

What to Use

- Pepper (as desired)

- Salt (as desired)

- Cream cheese (8 oz.)

- Salami (10 slices)

- Pickles (4 T)

What to Do

- Leave the cream cheese out until it reaches room temperature before placing it in a bowl and whipping it well.

- Spread the results onto a piece of plastic wrap so that it forms a .25-inch-thick square.

- Top the cream cheese with the pickles before topping the pickles with the salami in overlapping pieces.

- Place another layer of plastic wrap on the salami and press down firmly before flipping the entire thing over and peeling back the top plastic wrap layer from the cream cheese.

- Slowly roll the rectangle into a log shape, removing the plastic wrap as you go.

- Slice the log and serve.

Meatballs

Total Prep & Cooking Time: 40 minutes

Yields: 3 Servings

Nutrition Facts (per serving)

- Protein: 12 grams

- Net Carbs: 2 grams

- Fats: 7 grams

- Calories: 270

What to Use

- Pepper (as desired)

- Coconut oil (2 T)

- Salt (as desired)

- Italian sausage (1 lb.)

- Bacon (9 slices)

- Garlic (2 T minced)

- White onion (2 T diced)

- Oregano (1 T)

What to Do

- Ensure your over is set to 375F.

- Add the oil to the pan before placing it on the stove over a burner turned to a medium/high heat, add in the sausage and allow it to brown.

- Prepare a baking sheet by covering it in aluminum foil.

- Add all of the ingredients, with the exception of the bacon, and combine well.

- Form the results into 9 meatballs and warp a slice of bacon around each before placing them on the baking sheet. Place the meatballs in the oven for 30 minutes.

- Let the meatballs cool 5 minutes prior to serving.

Orange beef stew

Total Prep & Cooking Time: 8 hours and 10 minutes

Yields: 4 Servings

Nutrition Facts (per serving)

- Net carbs: 5 g

- Fats: 16 g

- Calories: 447

- Protein: 54 g

What to Use

- Salt (as needed)

- Pepper (as needed)

- Rutabagas (3 spiralized)

- Sage (1 T chopped fine)

- Thyme (1 T chopped fine)

- Rosemary (1 T chopped fine)

- Bay leaves (2)

- Cinnamon (2 tsp. ground)

- Water (4 cups)

- Balsamic vinegar (.25 cups)

- Orange juice (.5 cups)

- Orange zest (1 orange)

- Garlic (2 cloves minced)

- Celery (1 stalked diced)

- Carrot (1 diced)

- Onion (1 diced)

- Coconut oil (3 T)

- Beef stew meat (900 g cubed)

What to Do

- Add all of the ingredients except for the sage, thyme, rutabagas and rosemary to the slow cooker. Adjust the slow cooker temperature to low and leave it be, covered, for 8 hours.

- About 10 minutes prior to serving remove the bay leaves and add in the remaining ingredients.

Salad Ham Cups

Total Prep & Cooking Time: 38 minutes

Yields: 1 Serving

Nutrition Facts (per serving)

- Protein: 16 grams

- Net Carbs: 6 grams

- Fats: 12.9 grams

- Calories: 310

What to Use
- Cheddar cheese (.5 cups shredded)
- Ham (2 thin slices)
- Lettuce (shredded)
- Tomato (chopped)
- Egg (1 hard-boiled, sliced)

What to Do

- Ensure your oven is heated to 350F.
- Put muffin pan or custard cups on a cookie sheet.
- Put the 2 ham slices on top of an inverted muffin pan or custard cups in an x shape.
- Place the second custard on top of the first one, so the ham won't overcook. You are creating a "bowl" out of the ham.
- Cut off the excess ham. Leave about an inch. The ham will shrink.
- Bake 20 minutes.
- Once it has finished cooking, let it cool for 15 minutes.
- Remove top bowl. Cool. Remove bottom bowl when cool enough.

- Fill ham cup with the lettuce, egg, tomato and the cheese.
- Serve cold.

Chapter 5: Dinner Recipes

Quesadilla

Total Prep & Cooking Time: 23 minutes

Yields: 4 Servings

Nutrition Facts (per serving)

- Protein: 16 grams
- Net Carbs: 1 grams
- Fats: 43 grams
- Calories: 462

What to Use

- Almond meal (.75 c)
- Butter (5 T melted)
- Baking powder (1.5 tsp.)
- Splenda (1.5 tsp.)
- Oregano (.5 tsp.)
- Thyme (.5 tsp.)
- Garlic powder (.5 tsp.)
- Alfredo sauce (.5 c)
- Cheddar cheese (4 oz. shredded)

- Jarlsberg (2 oz.)

- Eggs (2 large)

What to Do

- Ensure your over is set to 450F.

- In a mixing bowl, combine the almond meal, baking powder, oregano, Splenda, thyme and garlic powder together and mix well.

- Warm the eggs in hot water before placing them in the dry mixture and adding in the melted butter as well. Combine thoroughly until the results form a dough.

- Prepare a pizza pan and add in the dough, taking care to spread it evenly. Place the pan in the oven and let everything cook about 7 minutes.

- Top with alfredo sauce and shredded cheese before returning the pizza pan back to the oven under the broil to brown for about 2 minutes.

Pork chops

Total Prep & Cooking Time: 45 minutes

Yields: 4 Servings

Nutrition Facts (per serving)

- Protein: 31 grams

- Net Carbs: 3 grams

- Fats: 25 grams

- Calories: 341

What to Use

- Pepper (as desired)

- Butter (4 T)

- Salt (as desired)

- Pork chops (4)

- Paprika (1 T)

- Garlic powder (1 tsp.)

- Onion powder (1 tsp.)

- Thyme leaves (.5 tsp.)

- Oregano leaves (.5 tsp.)

- Cumin (1 tsp.)

What to Do

- Mix together the pepper, cumin, salt, thyme leaves, cumin, onion powder, garlic powder and paprika and combine thoroughly.

- In a separate bowl melt the butter.

- Add 2 T coconut oil to the pan before placing it on the stove over a burner turned to a medium/high heat.

- Dip each porkchop in the butter, coat it thoroughly in the spice mixture and the cook each side about 4 minutes or until the chop's internal temperature reaches 150F.

- Serve hot and enjoy.

Keto burger

Total Prep & Cooking Time: 30 minutes

Yields: 3 Servings

Nutrition Facts (per serving)

- Protein: 22 grams

- Net Carbs: 1 gram

- Fats: 31 grams

- Calories: 385

What to Use

- Pepper (as desired)

- Coconut oil (2 T)

- Salt (as desired)

- Bacon (4 strips)

- Ground beef (1.5 lbs.)

- Eggs (2 large)

- Garlic powder (.5 tsp.)

- Onion powder (.5 tsp.)

- Worcestershire sauce (as desired)

- Cheddar cheese (8 oz.)

What to Do

- Combine the beef and eggs in a mixing bowl before adding in the spices and mixing well.

- Form the results into patties that weight 1.5 oz. each and topping each patty with .5 oz. of cheese. Combine two patties to form a single burger.

- Add the oil to the pan before placing it on the stove over a burner turned to a medium/high heat. Add one of the patties to the pan and cook for about 2 minutes or until it reaches your desired level of doneness.

- Separately, add the bacon to a frying pan and place the pan on top of a burner turned to a medium/high heat and cook until crisp.

- Top each burger with bacon prior to serving.

Flank steak

Total Prep & Cooking Time: 65 minutes

Yields: 6 Servings

Nutrition Facts (per serving)

- Protein: 54 grams

- Net Carbs: 3 grams

- Fats: 25 grams

- Calories: 470

What to Use

- Pepper (as desired)

- Salt (as desired)

- Flank steak (2)

- Spinach (16 oz.)

- Roasted peppers (7 oz. sliced)

- Bleu cheese (4 oz.)

- Almond flour (2 T)

- Egg yolk (1)

- Garlic powder (.5 tsp.)

- Onion powder (.5 tsp.)

What to Do

- Ensure your over is set to 400F.

- Start by working the steak from back to front and butterfly it, moving right to left as you go.

- Combine the remaining ingredients in a large mixing bowl and mix well.

- Cover the steak in the results from the bowl before rolling each steak up tightly and then wrapping it up using kitchen twine.

- Wrap each steak in plastic wrap before placing it in the refrigerator and allowing it to marinate for at least 60 minutes.

- Remove the plastic wrap and string from the steak and place it on a prepared baking sheet. Allow the steak to broil about 10 minutes, rotating at the halfway mark.

- Once the meat is cooked, remove the baking sheet from the oven, cover it in aluminum foil and let it rest 5 minutes before serving.

Spicy chicken

Total Prep & Cooking Time: 40 minutes

Yields: 4 Servings

Nutrition Facts (per serving)

- Protein: 44 grams

- Net Carbs: 4 grams

- Fats: 19 grams

- Calories: 281

What to Use

- Pepper (as desired)

- Salt (as desired)

- Chicken thighs (8, boneless, skinless)

- Chili and garlic sauce (2 T)

- Lime juice (3 T)

- Onion (1 small, chopped)

What to Do

- Ensure your over is set to 400F.

- Mix together salt and pepper as desired before using the results to thoroughly coat the chicken legs.

- Add the lime juice and chili sauce to a mixing bowl and combine thoroughly.

- Add the onion and chicken to the mixing bowl and coat well.

- Place all of the ingredients in a large skillet and then place the skillet in the oven for 35 minutes or until the chicken's internal temperature is 165F.

Brussel sprout surprise

Total Prep & Cooking Time: 45 minutes

Yields: 12 Servings

Nutrition Facts (per serving)

- Protein: 13 grams

- Net Carbs: 6 grams

- Fats: 39 grams

- Calories: 350

What to Use

- Brussels sprouts (2 lb. thinly sliced)

- Cheddar cheese (8 oz.)

- Thyme (2 tsp.)

- Garlic (2 T minced)

- Heavy cream (2 c)

- Parmesan cheese (4 oz. grated)

- Almond flour (1 c)

- Butter (2 T melted)

What to Do

- Ensure your over is set to 350F.

- Slice the brussels sprouts by hand or use a food processor to do the task in half the time.

- Add the sliced brussels sprouts to the mixing bowl before adding in the cheese, thyme and garlic and mixing well.

- Add the results to a casserole dish and spread them evenly.

- In another bowl combine the almond flour, parmesan cheese and butter and mix until it begins to form crumbles.

- Add the results to the top of the casserole and spread it evenly.

- Place the dish in the oven for about 30 minutes. You will know it is ready when the cheese begins to bubble and the crust is brown.

Chicken curry

Total Prep & Cooking Time: 40 minutes

Yields: 6 Servings

Nutrition Facts (per serving)

- Protein: 38 grams

- Net Carbs: 6 grams

- Fats: 17 grams

- Calories: 349

What to Use

- Pepper (as desired)

- Coconut oil (2 T)

- Salt (as desired)

- Chicken breast (4)

- Curry paste (1 packet)

- Water (1 c)

- Heavy cream (.5 c)

- Cauliflower (1 head)

What to Do

- Add the coconut oil and curry paste to a pan and mix well before adding in 1 c water. Place the pan on the stove on a low heat and allow it to simmer about 5 minutes before adding in the chicken and letting everything simmer about 20 minutes.

- While the chicken cooks prepare the cauliflower rice.

- Add the cream into the pan and let everything simmer an additional 5 minutes.

- Plate the cauliflower rice and top with chicken curry prior to serving.

Baked chicken

Total Prep & Cooking Time: 30 minutes

Yields: 4 Servings

Nutrition Facts (per serving)

- Protein: 63 grams

- Net Carbs: 3 grams

- Fats: 38 grams

- Calories: 527

What to Use

- Coconut oil (2 T)

- Chicken breasts (4)

- Bacon strips (4)

- Soy sauce (1 oz.)

- Ranch dressing (4 oz.)

- Green onions (3 chopped)

- Cheddar cheese (4 oz.)

What to Do

- Add the oil to a cast iron skillet before placing it on the stove over a burner turned to a high heat. Once the oil has melted, add in the chicken and let it cook about 10 minutes, flipping regularly. You will know it is ready when its internal temperature reaches 165F.

- As the chicken cooks, place the bacon in a frying pan before placing it on the stove over a burner turned to a medium/high heat. Allow the bacon to cook until it is crispy and then crumble it.

- Place the chicken in the baking dish and top it with ranch, soy sauce, cheese and green onions.

- Broil the baking dish for 3 minutes to brown the cheese prior to serving.

Cheddar biscuit burgers

Total Prep & Cooking Time: 45 minutes

Yields: 6 Servings

Nutrition Facts (per serving)

- Protein: 21 grams

- Net Carbs: 4 grams

- Fats: 43 grams

- Calories: 466

What to Use

- Cheddar cheese (6 slices + 4 oz.)

- Hamburger (1 lb.)

- Carbquik (2 c)

- Butter (2 oz. unsalted)

- Garlic powder (.5 tsp.)

- Salt (.5 tsp.)

- Heavy cream (.25 c)

- Water (.25 c)

What to Do

- Ensure your over is set to 450F.

- Add the Carbquik to a mixing bowl before adding in the butter and mixing until the results start to resemble dough.

- Add in the garlic powder, salt and cheese and mix well before adding in the liquid ingredients and forming proper dough.

- Split the results into six pieces before placing them on the prepared baking sheet.

- Place the baking sheet in the oven until the biscuits are a golden brown which should take about 8 minutes.

- As the biscuits bake, place the hamburger in the skillet before placing it on top of a burner set to a medium/high heat. Form the meat into patties as it browns.

- Let the biscuits cool 2 minutes before slicing each in half, adding a hamburger patty as well as a slice of cheese.

Pizza mushrooms

Total Prep & Cooking Time: 22 minutes

Yields: 3 Servings

Nutrition Facts (per serving)

- Protein: 19 grams

- Net Carbs: 4 grams

- Fats: 21 grams

- Calories: 276

What to Use

- Peperoni slice (12)

- Cheddar cheese (1.5 oz.)

- Monterey jack (1.5 oz.)

- Mozzarella (1.5 oz.)

- Spinach (9 leaves)

- Tomato (3 slices)

- Pizza seasoning (3 tsp.)

- Olive oil (to taste)

- Portobello mushrooms (3 large)

What to Do

- Start by making sure your oven is heated to 450F.

- Line a baking sheet using tinfoil and then set the mushrooms onto the baking sheet with the cap facing down before drizzling them in olive oil and seasoning as desired.

- Top with spinach, cheese and tomato before placing in the oven to bake for 6 minutes.

- Remove from the oven, add the pepperoni, and additional seasoning as needed before baking another 6 minutes.

Carnitas

Total Prep & Cooking Time: 8 hours and 15 minutes

Yields: 16 Servings

Nutrition Facts (per serving)

- Protein: 8 grams

- Net Carbs: 0grams

- Fats: 19 grams

- Calories: 265

What to Use

- Pepper (as desired)

- Water (1 c)

- Salt (as desired)

- Pork butt (8 lbs.)

- Bacon grease (2 T)

- Onion (1 large)

- Cumin (2 T)

- Thyme (2 T)

- Chili powder (2 T)

- Garlic (4 T minced)

What to Do

- Coat the pork with seasonings and rub well prior to placing it in the slow cooker. Add in the rest of the ingredients as well.

- Allow the slow cooker to cook, covered, for about 8 hours on a low heat.

Broccoli soup

Total Prep & Cooking Time: 10 minutes

Yields: 4 Servings

Nutrition Facts (per serving)

- Protein: 10 grams

- Net Carbs: 5 grams

- Fats: 23 grams

- Calories: 272

What to Use

- Pepper (as desired)

- Chicken bouillon (.5)

- Salt (as desired)

- Heavy cream (.25 c)

- Cream cheese 9.25 c)

- Sour cream (.25 c)

- Almond milk (.25 c)

- Cheddar cheese (4 oz.)

- Broccoli (7 oz.)

- Onion (.5)

What to Do

- Remove the broccoli florets and place them in a microwaveable bowl before adding a little water and microwaving for 3 minutes to allow the broccoli to steam.

- Add all of the liquid ingredients to a blender before adding in cheese, broccoli and onion. Break the bouillon cube over the top of the rest of the ingredients.

- Blend on the soup setting.

Shrimp and spinach

Total Prep & Cooking Time: 10 minutes

Yields: 2 Servings

Nutrition Facts (per serving)

- Fat: 24 grams

- Protein: 36 grams

- Net Carbs: 3 grams

- Calories: 301

What to Use

- Pepper (as desired)

- Coconut oil (1 T)

- Salt (as desired)

- Lemon (optional)

- Shrimp (20 large)

- Onion (.25 sliced)

- Garlic (3 cloves chopped)

- Butter (2 T)

- Parmesan cheese (.5 T)

- Spinach (2 handfuls)

What to Do

- Peel the shrimp and add them to cold water.

- Add the oil to the pan before placing it on the stove over a burner turned to a medium heat. Add in the shrimp and allow the m to cook until they are lightly pink. Remove them from the pan and set to one side.

- Add the garlic and onions to the pan and allow them to cook until the onions are translucent. Add in a dash of salt.

- Mix in the parmesan cheese, cream and butter and stir until smooth.

- Allow the sauce to thicken and cook about 2 minutes.

- Add the shrimp back into the pan and allow them to cook all the way through which should take about 3 minutes. Take care not to overcook the shrimp or else it will become tough and dry.

- Remove the sauce and the shrimp from the pan and add in the spinach. Allow the spinach to cook about 45 seconds.

- Plate the spinach then top with the shrimp and a squeeze of lemon.

Tuna Casserole

Total Prep & Cooking Time: 40 minutes

Yields: 2 Servings

Nutrition Facts (per serving)

- Net Carbs: 4.5 grams

- Protein: 21 grams

- Fats: 33 grams

- Calories: 459

What to Use

- Cheddar cheese (4 oz. shredded)

- Celery (1 stalk, hashed fine)

- Pepper (as desired)

- Salt (as desired)

- Onion (2 T chopped fine)

- Heavy cream (.75 c)

- Chicken broth (.5 c)

- Butter (2 T)

- Mushrooms (3 oz. sliced)

- Green beans (16 oz. French cut)

- Tuna (12 oz. drained)

What to Do

- Add the green beans to a medium-sized pot and cook well before draining.

- Add the onion, mushrooms, celery and butter to a pan before placing it on the stove over a burner turned to a medium heat and let everything cook about 5 minutes.

- Add in the broth and let it boil before turning the heat
  down and allowing it to simmer until it has reduced
  50 percent. Add in the cream and turn the heat back
  up to allow the pot to boil.

- Reduce the heat and allow the sauce to thicken once
  more, stirring regularly.

- Season as desired before putting the tuna and
  mushroom mixture into the green beans.

- Preheat the oven to 400F.

- Add in the cheese and mix thoroughly.

- Add the results to a 2 quart casserole dish.

- Place the casserole dish in the oven and allow it to
  cook about 15 minutes.

Chapter 6: Snacks Recipes

Cauliflower tots

Total Prep & Cooking Time: 45 minutes

Yields: 6 Servings

Nutrition Facts (per serving)

- Protein: 11.6 grams

- Net Carbs: 4.8 grams

- Fats: 20.7 grams

- Calories: 205

What to Use

- Pepper (as desired)

- Salt (as desired)

- Cauliflower (1 medium, cut into florets)

- Water (.25 c)

- Cheddar cheese (1 c shredded)

- Almond meal (.75 c)

- Bacon (8 slices chopped)

- Green chilies (7 oz.)

- Jalapeno slices (2 T)

- Eggs (2 large)

-

What to Do

- Ensure your over is set to 400F.

- Place the cauliflower in the food processor and process well. Add the results to a medium-sized saucepan and then add in enough water to steam it properly. Add the pan to a burner turned to a low heat and allow it to steam about 10 minutes.

- Drain the cauliflower and remove any excess moisture.

- Prepare a mini-muffin pan that has 24 mini-muffin cups.

- In a large mixing bowl combine all of the ingredients and mix well.

- Divide the results evenly within the muffin tin and press down to ensure each cup is well-compacted.

- Place the tin in the oven for about 25 minutes or until you can push a toothpick through the center tot and remove it cleanly.

- Let them cool for 5 minutes on the dot as any long will ensure they stick to the pan.

Flaxseed Muffins

Total Prep & Cooking Time: 25 minutes

Yields: 6 Servings

Nutrition Facts (per serving)

- Carbs: 1.2 grams

- Protein: 4.2 grams

- Fat: 9.4 grams

- Calories: 120

What to Use

- Flaxseed (1 c ground)

- Erythritol (.3 c)

- Baking powder (.5 T)

- Cinnamon (1 T)

- Salt (.5 tsp.)

- Flaxseed eggs (3 large)

- Vanilla extract (1 tsp.)

- Coconut oil (3 T)

- Almond milk (2 T)

- Red currants (.5 c)

What to Do

- Ensure your over is set to 350F.

- Prepare a muffin tin by greasing it with coconut oil.

- Add all of the dry ingredients to a mixing bowl

- Separately, add all of the wet ingredients to a mixing bowl and then combine the two bowls and mix well. Add in the red currants and ensure they are evenly dispersed.

- Add the batter evenly to the muffin tins, taking care to leave space for the muffins to rise.

- Place the muffin tin in the oven to bake about 15 minutes.

- Let the muffins cool 5 minutes prior to removing from the tin.

Hotdogs wrapped in bacon

Total Prep & Cooking Time: 50 minutes

Yields: 6 Servings

Nutrition Facts (per serving)

- Protein: 17 grams

- Net Carbs: 0 grams

- Fat: 35 grams

- Calories: 380

What to Use

- Pepper (as desired)

- Salt (as desired)

- Garlic powder (.5 tsp.)

- Onion powder (.5 tsp.)

- Sharp cheddar (2 oz.)

- Hot dogs (6 wieners)

- Bacon (12 slices)

What to Do

- Ensure your over is set to 400F.

- Cut the hotdogs lengthwise about halfway through each, take care to ensure you don't cut all the way through the wiener.

- Slice the cheese into comparable strips and then stuff each wiener. Take care to ensure no cheese hangs over the edge.

- Wrap each hot dog completely in bacon, each wiener should require 2 pieces of bacon. Wrap each wiener tightly and use toothpicks to hold everything together if needed.

- When all the dogs are wrapped place them on a wire rack that is itself placed on top of a cookie sheet. Season the wieners with salt, pepper, onion powder and garlic powder.

- Place the wieners in the oven for about 40 minutes or until the bacon is noticeably crisp. You can then broil for a few extra minutes as desired.

- Remove the toothpicks prior to serving.

Bacon and brussels sprouts

Total Prep & Cooking Time: 35 minutes

Yields: 4 Servings

Nutrition Facts (per serving)

- Net Carbs: 4 grams

- Protein: 15 grams

- Fat: 21 grams

- Calories: 310

What to Use

- Pepper (as desired)

- Coconut oil (2 T)

- Salt (as desired)

- Brussels sprouts (1 lb. halved)

What to Do

- Ensure your over is set to 375F.

- Add the brussels sprouts to a greased baking sheet and top each with the coconut oil. Mix together the salt and pepper and then top the brussels sprouts with the mixture.

- Place the baking sheet in the oven for about half an hour. Remove the sheet from the oven after 15 minutes and shake the sprouts to mix things up a bit.

- As the sprouts are cooking fry the bacon until it is crispy.

- After the bacon has finished cooking, crumble it.

- Plate the sprouts and top with bacon prior to serving.

Vegan crackers

Total Prep & Cooking Time: 15 minutes

Yields: 2 Servings

Nutrition Facts (per serving)

- Calories: 156

- Protein: 6.1 g

- Carbohydrates: 1.2 g

- Fat: 12.4 g

What to Use

- Pepper (as desired)

- Spices and herbs (as desired)

- Salt (as desired)

- Water (1 c)

- Psyllium husk fiber (2 tsp.)

- Hemp seeds (.25 c)

- Sesame seeds (.5 c)

- Flax seeds (.5 c)

What to Do

- Add all of the ingredients to a food processor or blender and process or blend well until the results achieve a flour-like texture.

- Add the flour to a mixing bowl before slowing adding in the water while stirring slowly. Continue stirring until the water has been completely absorbed.

- Allow the results 5 minutes to firm up before spreading the results on a pair of dehydrator trays. When spreading the mixture, aim for a thickness of less than .25 in.

- Dehydrate the chips overnight at 115F. Wait 8 hours and then flip the chips over before dehydrating for an addition 4 hours.

- Place the chips in an airtight container and they will last about 7 days.

Coleslaw

Total Prep & Cooking Time: 15 minutes

Yields: 2 Servings

Nutrition Facts (per serving)

- Calories: 84

- Protein: 2.6 g

- Carbohydrates: 4.5 g

- Fat: 5.8 g

What to Use

- Coconut oil (1 T)

- Garlic (.5 tsp. minced)

- Ginger (.5 tsp. grated)

- Sesame oil (1 T)

- Tamari (1 T)

- Rice wine vinegar (1 T)

- Sesame seeds (2 T)

- Carrots (.25 c shredded)

- Scallions (2 sliced thin)

- Green cabbage (2 c shredded)

- Red cabbage (2 c shredded)

What to Do

- Mix up the ingredients used for the dressing then set apart for their flavors to fuse.

- Mix the other salad ingredients in a large bowl and toss the vegetables with the dressing.

- Garnish the meal by sprinkling the sesame seeds on top.

- Serve and enjoy!

Mini nachos

Total Prep & Cooking Time: 25 minutes

Yields: 4 Servings

Nutrition Facts (per serving)

- Net Carbs: 2.2 grams

- Protein: 26.7 grams

- Fats: 24.5 grams

- Calories: 367

What to Use

- Pepper (as desired)

- Salt (as desired)

- Oregano (.5 tsp.)

- Red pepper flakes (.25 tsp.)

- Paprika (1 tsp.)

- Ground beef (16 oz.)

- Garlic powder (1 tsp.)

- Mini peppers(16 oz. halved, seeded)

- Cumin (1 tsp. ground)

- Sharp cheddar (1.5 c)

- Chili powder (1 T)

- Tomato (.5 c chopped)

What to Do

- Combine all of the seasonings in a mixing bowl.

- Place the meat in a pan before placing the ban on the stove on top of a burner turned to a medium heat. As the meat browns make sure to break it up, mixing in the spices as you do.

- Ensure your oven is heated to 400F.

- Place the peppers on a prepared baking sheet and coat them with the beef mixture before topping them with cheese.

- Place the baking sheet in the oven for about 10 minutes.

- Top with the remaining toppings prior to serving.

Kale and artichoke dip

Total Prep & Cooking Time: 4 hours and 5 minutes

Yields: 20 Servings

Nutrition Facts (per serving)

- Fiber: 2 g

Net carbs: 5 g

- Fats: 4 g

- Calories: 98

- Protein: 6 g

What to Use

- Salt (as needed)

- Pepper (as needed)

- Low fat mayonnaise (.25 c)

- Light sour cream (.75 c)

- Greek yogurt (1 c plain)

- Mozzarella cheese (1 c shredded)

- Parmesan cheese (1 c)

- Kale (10 oz. chopped)

- Spinach (10 oz. chopped)

- Artichoke hearts (28 oz. drained)

- Onion (.5 diced)

- Garlic (2 cloves chopped)

What to Do

- Add the onion, artichokes and garlic to a food processor until it begins to form a paste.

- Place each ingredient into your slow cooker. Adjust the slow cooker temperature to high and leave it be, covered, for about 4 hours.

- Season as desired prior to serving.

Pecan maple bites

Total Prep & Cooking Time: 55 minutes

Yields: 6 Servings

Nutrition Facts (per serving)

- Protein: 17 grams

- Net Carbs: 3.2 grams

- Fat: 25 grams

- Calories: 180

What to Use – Maple syrup

- Coconut oil (2.25 tsp.)

- Water (.75 c)

- Erythritol (.25 c powdered)

- Unsalted butter (1 T)

- Maple extract (2 tsp.)

- Vanilla extract (.5 tsp.)

- Xanthan gum (.25 tsp.)

- Cinnamon (.5 tsp.)

What to Use – Bits

- Pecan halves (2 c)

- Almond flour (1 c)

- Golden flaxseed meal (.5 c)

- Shredded coconut (.5 c)

- Maple syrup (.25 c)

- Coconut oil (.5 c)

- Liquid stevia (.25 tsp.)

What to Do - Syrup

- In a microwaveable container, combine the xanthan gum, coconut oil and butter and mix well. Microwave the container for 40 seconds.

- In a spice grinder add the cinnamon and erythritol and grind well.

- Add the results to a small bowl before adding in .75 c water as well as the maple and vanilla extracts and combine thoroughly.

- Microwave for another 40 seconds and stir well.

- Allow the syrup to cool prior to use.

- This recipe will make 1 c of liquid.

What to Do – Bites

- Ensure your oven is heated to 350F.

- Place the pecan halves on a baking tray covered in aluminum foil before placing the baking tray in the oven for approximately 6 minutes.

- Place the baked pecan halves in a Ziploc bag and crush them using a rolling pin.

- Combine the almond flour, flaxseed meal and shredded coconut together in a mixing bowl and then mix in the crushed pecans.

- Add in the coconut oil, maple syrup and liquid stevia and mix until the mixture creates a dough.

- Add the dough to a casserole dish before placing the dish in the oven for 20 minutes.

- Refrigerate the for 60 minutes prior to cutting and serving.

Almond butter cups

Total Prep & Cooking Time: 60 minutes

Yields: 12 Servings

Nutrition Facts (per serving)

- Net Carbs: 3.5 grams

- Protein: 3 grams

- Fats: 28 grams

- Calories: 238

What to Use

- Coconut oil (2 T)

- Salt (.25 tsp.)

- Agave syrup (.25 c)

- Coconut oil (2 T melted)

- Almond butter (.5 c)

- Semisweet chocolate (12 oz. finely chopped)

What to Do

- Prepare a muffin tray by lining it with plastic liners.

- Place the chocolate into a small pan before placing the pan on top of the stove over a burner set to a low heat and stir while it melts.

- After the chocolate, has melted most of the way, remove the pan from heat and keep stirring until the remainder has melted.

- Add 1 ½ tsp. of chocolate to each muffin liner and ensure it covers have an inch of space. The chocolate should be as even as possible before you place it in the refrigerator to cool for 15 minutes or until it has solidified.

- While the chocolate cools, take a small bowl and add in the salt, agave syrup, coconut oil and almond butter and mix well, the results should be completely smooth which may require the use of a small pastry brush.

- Add the results to the top of the chocolate in the lined muffin tin and smooth it out as best as you can before adding an extra 1 tsp. of chocolate to the top of each c.

- Top with sea salt and let them refrigerate an additional 30 minutes to ensure they harden properly.

Vanilla Fat Bomb

Total Prep & Cooking Time: 10 minutes

Yields: 2 Servings

Nutrition Facts (per serving)

- Protein: 16 grams

- Net Carbs: 2 grams

- Fats: 25.3 grams

- Calories: 301

What to Use

- Cream Cheese (10 oz. softened

- Butter (.6 c softened)

- Swerve (.6 c)

- Vanilla (.5 tsp.)

What to Do

- Line a baking sheet using wax paper.

- Combine all of the ingredients with the help of a hand mixer.

- Separate the results into 1 tablespoon servings when spacing them on the baking sheet.

- Let the bombs freeze for 60 minutes before removing them from the wax paper.

Cinnamon bars

Total Prep & Cooking Time: 10 minutes

Yields: 2 Servings

Nutrition Facts (per serving)

- Protein: 5 grams

- Net Carbs: 2.4 grams

- Fats: 21.8 grams

- Calories: 202

What to Use

- Creamed coconut (.6 c chunked)
- Cinnamon (1 tsp. divided)
- Coconut oil (1.25 T)
- Almond butter (1.25 T + 1 T)

What to Do

- Fill a baking dish using muffin liners.
- Mix the coconut cream and cinnamon together and then add the mix to the muffin liners.
- Separately, mix the 1 tablespoon of almond butter as well as the coconut oil and add to the muffin liners as well.
- Freeze before topping with the remaining ingredients.

Vanilla coffee cookies

Total Prep & Cooking Time: 27 minutes

Yields: 10 Servings

Nutrition Facts (per serving)

- Protein: 3.9 grams
- Net Carbs: 1.4 grams

- Fats: 17.1 grams

- Calories: 167

What to Use

- Liquid stevia (17 drops)

- Cinnamon (.25 tsp.)

- Kosher salt (.5 tsp.)

- Baking soda (.5 tsp.)

- Vanilla extract (1.5 tsp.)

- Instant coffee grounds (1 T + 1 tsp.)

- Eggs (2 large)

- Erythritol (.3 c)

- Unsalted butter (.5 c)

- Almond flour (1.5 c)

What to Do

- Start by making sure your oven is heated to 350 degrees F.

- Combine the cinnamon, salt, baking soda, coffee grounds and almond flour together in a mixing bowl.

- In a pair of separate bowls, separate the egg yolks from the egg whites.

- In yet another bowl, place your butter and beat it thoroughly before mixing in the erythritol and beating some more until the mixture is nearly white.

- Add in the egg yolks and mix well.

- Add in 50 percent of the flour and coffee mixture and mix well before adding in the liquid stevia as well of the vanilla extract and then finally the rest of the almond flour.

- Beat the whites of the eggs until they begin to form peaks and then add the results to the mixing bowl and mix thoroughly.

- Form the dough into 10 cookies on a cookie sheet before placing the sheet in the oven and letting it bake for 12 minutes.

- Let the cookies cool for 10 minutes prior to eating.

Conclusion

Thanks for making it through to the end of *Ketogenic Diet Book for Beginners*, let's hope it was informative and able to provide you with all of the tools you need to achieve your goals, whatever it is that they may be. Just because you've finished this book doesn't mean there is nothing left to learn on the topic, and expanding your horizons is the only way to find the mastery you seek.

When switching to the keto diet it is important that you have appropriate expectations when it comes to the weight loss that awaits you. While the keto diet is a great way to help your body burn fat like never before, this doesn't mean that you are immediately going to drop 10 pounds overnight. It is important to keep in mind that it will take some time for your body to ramp up its fat loss mechanisms which means that expecting too much too soon is only going to lead to severe disappointment. What's worse, building up unreasonable expectations might keep you from living up to your potential because not living up to some arbitrary goal might be all it takes for you to fall off the keto diet for good. Avoid these potential pitfalls entirely by focusing on sticking to the keto diet and letting the weight loss take care of itself.

Additionally, it is important to always discuss any major dietary changes with a healthcare professional to ensure you don't accidentally end up doing more harm than good.
Finally, if you found this book useful in anyway, a review on Amazon is always appreciated!

Description

The ketogenic diet is a great way to help jump-start your body's natural fat loss potential and help you to look and feel better than you have in years in the process. If you are interested in learning more, then the *Ketogenic Diet Book for Beginners* is the book you have been waiting for.

Getting started with the keto diet successfully does require some hard work, however, which is the chapters inside will discuss everything you need to know in order to move forward with this new healthy lifestyle choice successfully. First, you will learn all about what sets the keto diet apart from the pack as well as what you will need in order to follow it yourself. Next, you will learn all about the best ways to get started with keto diet yourself, as well as plenty of tips for dealing with the dreaded keto flu. From there you will find plenty of breakfast, lunch, dinner and snack recipes to help you start off on your new lifestyle choice on the right foot.

So, what are you waiting for? Your body can naturally burn fat for fuel, all it needs is your help, all it needs is for you to buy this book today!

Inside you will find recipes like

- Chia seed pudding

- Pizza chicken

- Lemon chicken with asparagus

- Brussel sprout surprise

- Tuna Casserole

- Hotdogs wrapped in bacon

- Cauliflower tots

- Almond butter cups

- Vanilla coffee cookies

- ***And more...***